Body Scrubs:

35 Natural DIY Scrubs for Body and Face for Radiant and Youthful Skin

Table of content:

Introduction

Want to make your own scrubs

You have seen many scrubs in the store for your body and face. You have seen the results of using them, but the problem you would like to save money by making your own. You've looked all over the internet to find information on how to make scrubs on your own, but the flood of information is difficult to parse and find just what you are looking for in order to get started. In this book, I use my over twenty years of natural health experience to walk you through everything you will need to get started and eventually make your own. I will teach you the basics and leave you feeling like you can start making your own recipes and using them.

You're ready to get started...

By purchasing this book, you are ready to get started on a new way to take care of your skin and your body. This book will walk you through the steps and show you:

• What scrubs are and the different types.
• What essential oils are and how to use them
• The best ways to combine the essential oils
• Recipes with step-by-step instructions on how to make and store the scrubs

I will present the information in a fashion that is easy to understand without leaving you with more questions. I will walk you through every step of the process. So, if you're ready to get started, let's get to it.

Chapter 1 - What is a scrub?

We've seen all manner and types of scrubs to exfoliate and help to heal skin. Scrubs can smooth rough spots on elbows and knees. They can also help to lightly scrub off dead skin from the face and other areas well. It can also moisturize your skin as well.

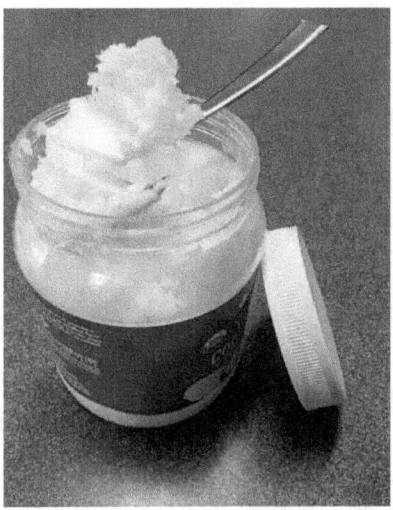

What you need...

There are a few simple things you will need to get started on your new hobby.

• Glass mixing bowls: You will need two of these to keep the dry ingredients separate from the wet ones until you are ready to mix them.

• Measuring cups: This is for measuring the sugar and other ingredients you will need.

• Wooden or glass spoons for mixing

• Airtight containers to store your scrubs

- Oils to mix into your scrubs

- Sugar, white or brown, preferably organic

- Essential oils

- Gloves to protect your hands while mixing

The oils

Before we get into the essential oils and safety, you need other oils, carrier oils to act as a base for the essential oil blends. Here is a list that you can use interchangeably or even mix together.

Coconut Oil

This oil is used more often than others when making scrubs because of the different fatty acids that tone and smooth skin.

It is solid at room temperature, which makes it good when placing the rub. It will melt when it comes in contact with the skin.

Olive Oil

This oil is also good for the skin because of its high concentration of vitamin E.

Almond Oil

Usually used for other preparations, I have found its very light, almost non-existent fragrance, makes it perfect for scrubs.

It is rich in protein and good for all types of skin. It also helps if you are suffering from dry and itchy and skins.

Apricot Kernel

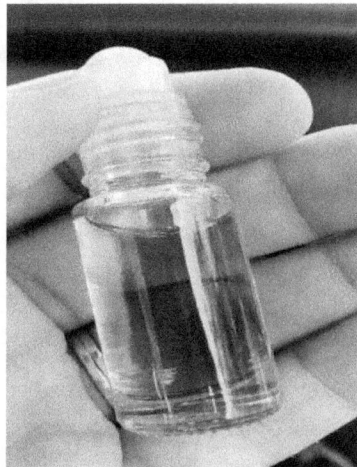

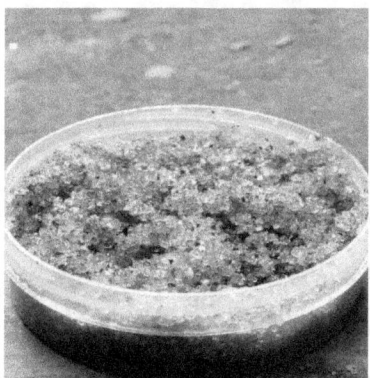

This is another light oil. It is used for sensitive skin. So, if you experience irritation from the other oils or are allergic to almonds, it is a good alternative because of its vitamin and mineral content.

Essential Oils

There are a list of essential oils you can use for your skin to help it look younger and healthier.

Cautions and Care

An essential oil is the most potent form of any plant; however, there are a few things you need to know about essential oils before you begin to use them.

1. Can cause contact dermatitis when used un-diluted. There are websites out there that will tell it is alright not to dilute the oils. This is false.

2. If you are not sure whether your skin will have a reaction to the use of certain essential oils, you can go to your nearest store that sells them and ask for a patch test. This will help you determine which essential oils will be alright for you to use.

3. Store the essential oils in a cool, dry place. Many essential oils are very light and will evaporate when exposed to heat.

4. Store your scrubs in tightly lidded dark glass containers to prevent light from entering and possibly heating up the mixture.

5. Scrubs have the same shelf life as the sugar you used to make them. It is best not to keep them longer than that. For maximum potency, use them after letting sit overnight in the container.

6. Do not apply scrubs to cracked, raw skin or open wounds. It will irritate the area to which it is applied.

The listc v

Bergamot, *Citrus bergamia*
This one is good for treating cold sores as well as acne, and greasy skin.

Cedarwood, Texas, *Juniperus ashei*
This is the first of two types of Cedarwood that are used for skin issues. This help with oily skin, it also helps with acne, eczema, psoriasis.

Cedarwood, Virginian, *Juniperus virginiana*
This essential oil is also good for the same things of its relative. The difference is, being a different genus, it can be gentler than the Texas version.

Chamomile, Roman, *Chamaemelum nobile*
This is an especially good essential oil for acne, eczema, light rashes, dermatitis, and inflammations.

Clary Sage, *salvia sclarea*
This is an essential oil that is good for regulating oily skin, and also helping to reduce swelling and fight acne. It's good for wrinkles, too.

Clove Bud, *Syzygium armaticum*
This is good for stubborn acne.

Galbanum, *Ferula galbaniflua*
This helps to heal scar tissue, tones skin, wrinkles as well as acne.

Geranium, *Pelargonium graveolens*
This essential oil is excellent for speeding the healing of broken capillaries, acne, burns, helps to unclog pores, and balances an oily complexion.

Grapefruit, *Citrus x paradisi*

This essential oil helps to tone and reduce sagging in skin and skin. It helps to unclog pore and regulate skin. It is also good for acne.

Helichrysum, *Helichrysum angutifolium*

This essential oil can help with inflammations of the skin caused by rosacea and puffiness around the eyes, chin and other problem areas. It has also been used to help treat acne, dermatitis, eczema, and age spots and blemishes for pinched zits.

Juniper, *Juniperus communis*

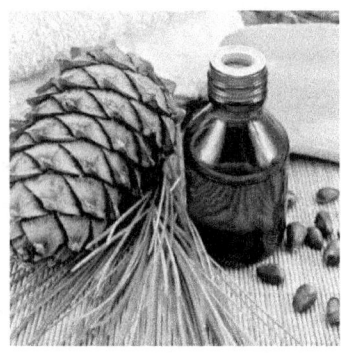

This essential oil is used to help treat acne breakouts and existing pimples. It has also been used to help treat skin conditions such as dermatitis and rosacea. It is also a skin toner.

Lavender, *Lavendula angustifolia*

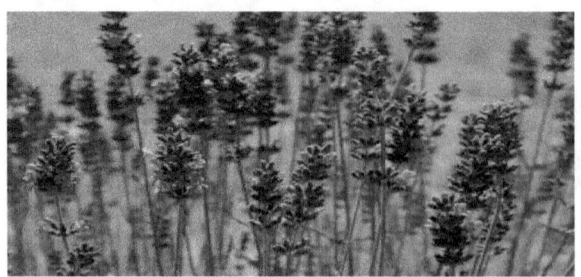

Combining Essential Oils

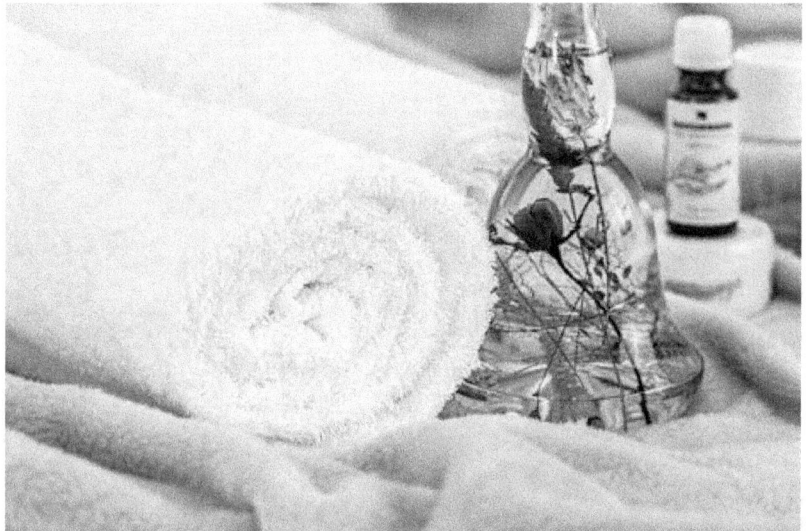

There are three types of essential oils:

Light
Medium,
And heavy.

These are usually known as "notes". When combining them, you will generally use more of the light and medium than you would the heavy. Making blends is usually in small batches, one tablespoon at a time. Here is a standard blend measure:

1 tbsp+6 drops of essential oil.

Now, obviously making scrubs, especially in large batches, would mean you're using more than one tablespoon in most cases. So, here is another guide.

Base recipe for Sugar scrubs:

1/2 cup sugar, white or brown
1/2 cup oil
50 Drops essential oil blend
• Blend the oils first.
• Stir the sugar into the oil blend.

Instructions for use:

Place thins layer of the scrub on the face, elbows, knees, or any non-sensitive part of the body. Scrub the area in small circles. Rinse with warm water and soap.

Now, that we've got the basics out of the way. Let's get on with the recipes.

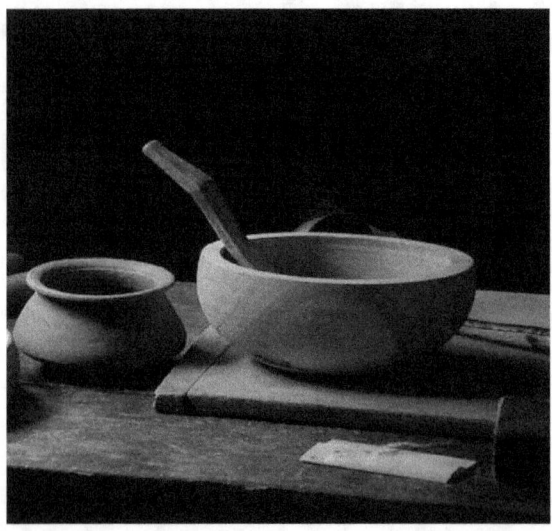

Chapter 2 - The Recipes

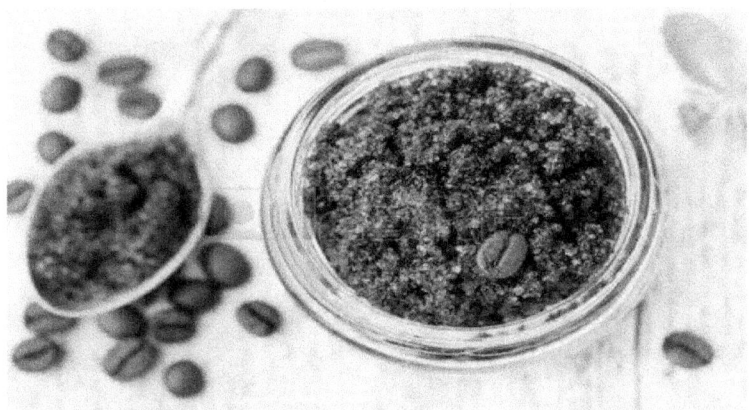

1. Oily Skin I

1/4 Cup Coconut Oil

1/4 Cup Almond Oil

20 Drops Lavender Essential Oil

10 Drops Tea Tree Essential Oil

10 Drops Texas Cedarwood Essential Oil

10 Drops Clary Sage Essential Oil

2. Oily Skin II

1/4 Cup Almond Oil

1/4 Cup Olive Oil

20 Drops Geranium Essential Oil

10 Drops Juniper Essential Oil

10 Drops Palmarosa Essential Oil

10 Drops Roman Chamomile Essential Oil

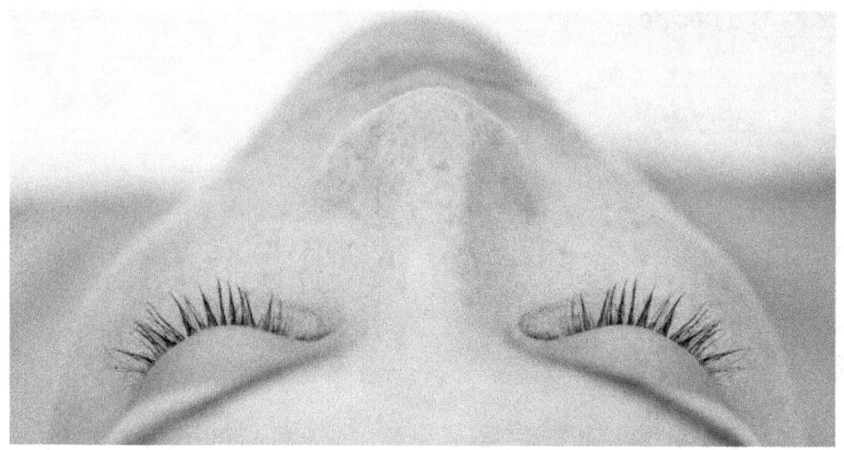

No doubt many of you have seen me type both "greasy" and "oily skin". There is a slight difference between the two. Oily skin tends to maintain a sheen on your face which is steady throughout the day, making you constantly check your makeup to cover those "shiny spots". Greasy skin is a more severe form of oily skin. Greasy skin produces more oils, making it impossible to go through a day and not have to wash your face to get rid of the excess oils.

There are ways of combatting oily/greasy skin besides washing your face and using scrubs:

1. Moisturize your skin. I know this may seem like you are adding oils to an already oily situation, but a nice and light moisturizer can prevent your skin from pulling in or producing too much oil to keep itself from drying out.

2. Keep a food diary. Even though many may say what you eat will not affect your skin, not all body chemistry is the same. One person can eat as much chocolate as they want and never have a skin problem while another, figuratively, breaks out just by looking at the confection.

3. Don't overdo it with washing your face. Keeping you face clean is a good idea, but if you are washing your face more than twice a day, you may be washing it too much. Your skin needs to produce some natural oils to maintain a pH balance, and when you are constantly washing your skin, you're forcing it to over compensate.

3. Greasy skin I

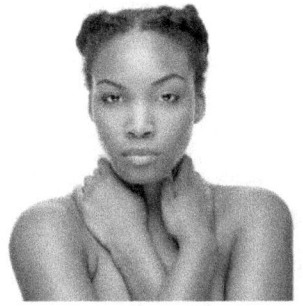

1/2 Cups Almond Oil

20 Drops Bergamot Essential Oil

10 Drops Lime Essential Oil

5 Drops Sandalwood Essential Oil

15 Drops Myrtle Essential Oil

10 Drops Virginia Cedarwood Essential Oil

4. Greasy Skin II

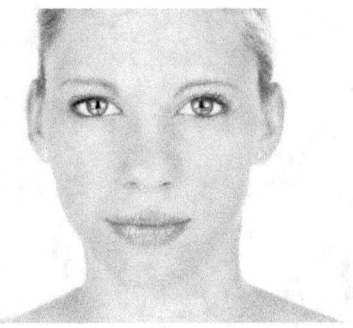

1/2 Cup Apricot Oil

20 Drops Lime Essential Oil

10 Drops Peppermint Essential Oil

10 Drops Patchouli Essential Oil

10 Drops Rosewood Essential Oil

5. Skin Toner

1/2 Cup Coconut Oil
20 Drops Grapefruit Essential oil
10 Drops Violet Essential Oil
10 Drops Juniper Essential Oil
10 Drops Rosewood Patchouli Essential Oil

6. Sensitive Skin Toner

1/4 Cup Almond Oil
1/4 Cup Olive Oil
20 Drops Lavender Essential Oil
10 Drops Rosewood Essential Oil
10 Drops Violet Essential Oil
10 Drops Ylang Ylang Essential Oil

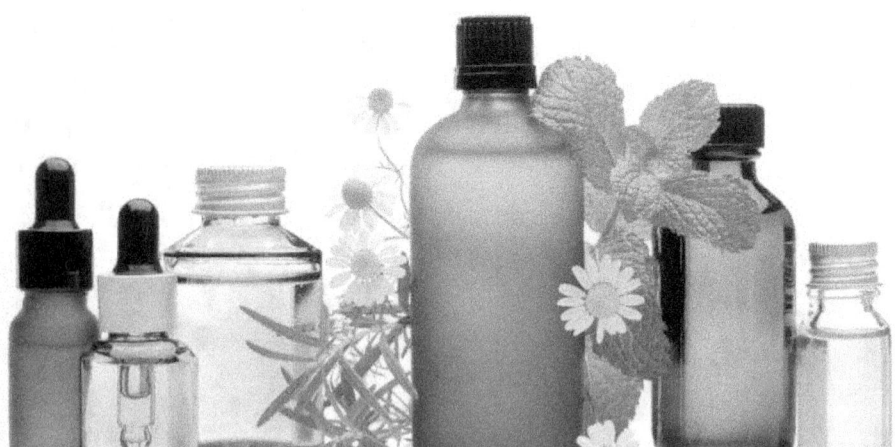

7. Dry Skin I

1/4 Cup Olive Oil
1/4 Coconut Oil
20 Drops Palmarosa Essential Oil
15 Drops Lavender Essential Oil
15 Drops Peppermint Essential Oil

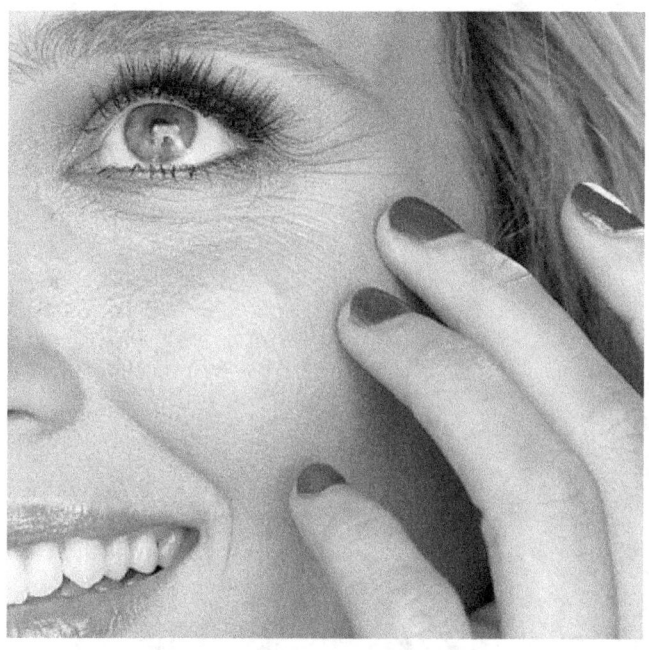

8. Dry Skin II

1/2 Cup Coconut Oil
15 Drops Rosewood Essential Oil
15 Drops Naouli Essential Oil
10 Drops Patchouli Essential Oil
10 Drops Vetiver Essential Oil

9. Toning I

1/4 Cup Coconut Oil
1/4 Cup Apricot Oil
15 Drops Grapefruit Essential Oil
15 Drops Juniper Essential Oil
10 Drops Virginia Cedarwood Essential Oil
10 Drops Sandalwood Essential Oil

10. Toning II

1/2 Coconut Oil
20 Drops Grapefruit Essential Oil
15 Drops Lavender Essential Oil
15 Drops Galbanum Essential Oil

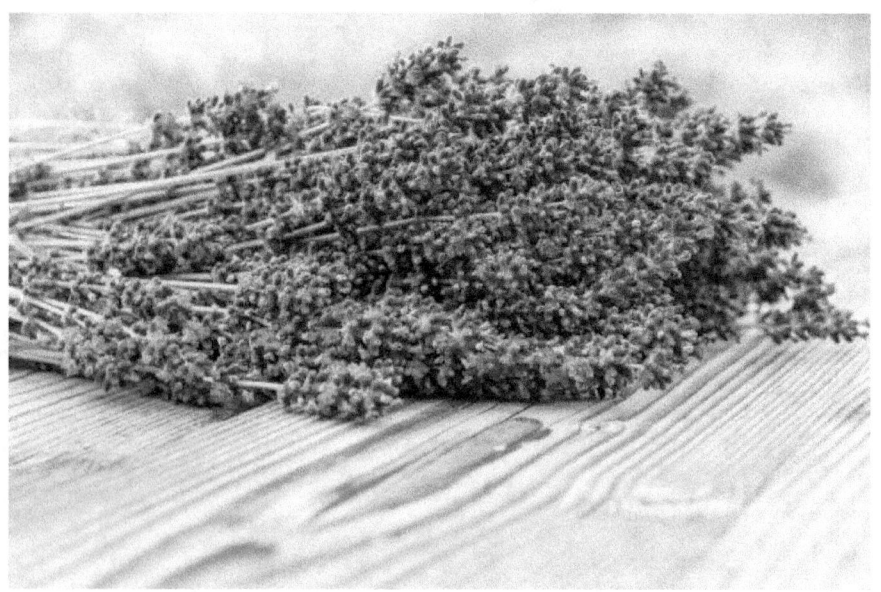

11. Wrinkle Scrub

1/4 Cup Coffee dry coffee grounds
1/4 Cup Cacao Ground
1/2 Cup Coconut Oil
20 Drops Lavender Essential Oil
10 Drops Clary Sage Essential Oil
10 Drops Palmarosa
10 Drops Grapefruit

12. Toning Scrub III

1/2 Cup Coffee Grounds
1/2 Cup Coconut Oil
20 Drops Grapefruit Essential Oil
15 Drops Roman Chamomile Essential Oil
15 Drops Peppermint Essential Oil

13. Soothing I

1/4 Cup Olive Oil
1/4 Cup Almond Oil
20 Drops Geranium Essential Oil
15 Drops Galbanum Essential Oil
15 Drops Vetiver Essential Oil

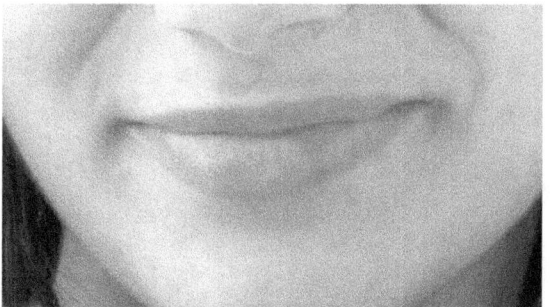

14. Soothing II

1/4 Cup Coconut Oil
1/4 Cup Almond Oil
15 Drops Violet
15 Drops Ylang Ylang
10 Drops Myrtle Essential Oil
10 Drops Rosewood Essential Oil

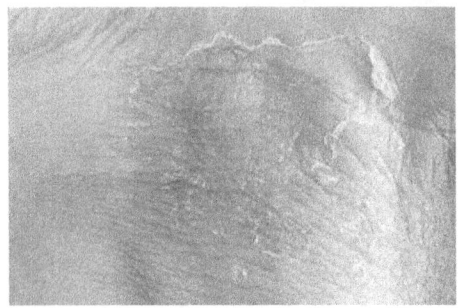

15. Eczema I

(Don't rub into broken skin)
1/2 Cup Coconut Oil
20 Drops Lavender Essential Oil
15 Drops Rosewood Essential Oil
5 Drops Sandalwood Oil
10 Drops Patchouli Essential Oil

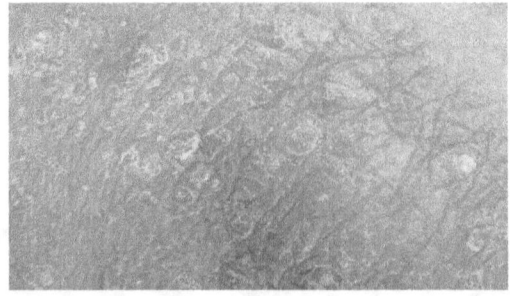

16. Eczema II

(Don't rub on broken skin)
1/2 Almond Oil
15 Drops Chamomile Essential Oil
15 Drops Lavender Essential Oil
10 Drops Violet Essential Oil
10 Drops Juniper Essential Oil

17. General Use I

1/2 Cup Olive Oil
10 Drops Lavender Essential Oil
10 Drops Grapefruit Essential Oil
10 Drops Rosewood Essential Oil
10 Drops Chamomile Essential Oil
10 Drops Myrtle Essential Oil

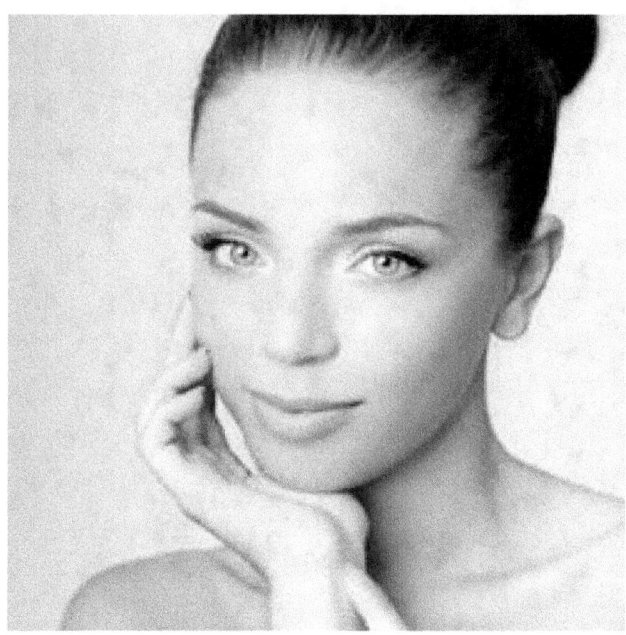

18. General Use II

1/2 Cup Coconut Oil
15 Drops Lavender Essential Oil
10 Drops Peppermint Essential Oil
10 Drops Palmarosa Essential Oil
5 Drops Clove Essential Oil
10 Drops Galbanum Essential Oil

19. Refining I

1/8 Cup Olive Oil
1/8 Cup Coconut Oil
1/4 Cup Almond Oil
15 Drops of Geranuim Essential Oil
10 Drops of Patchouli Essential oil
15 Drops of Lime Essential Oil
10 Drops Peppermint Essential Oil

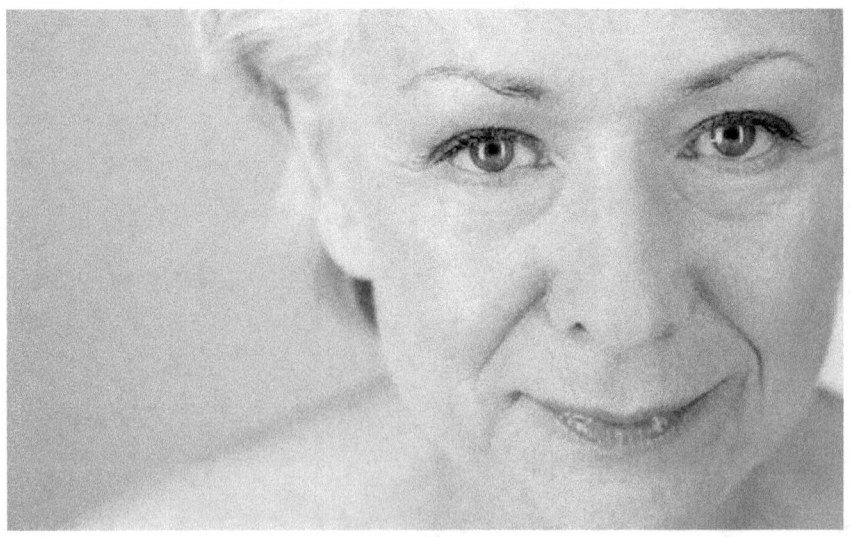

20. Refining II Mature Skin

This one is recommended for older skin.

1/4 Cup Olive Oil

1/4 Cup Coconut Oil

20 Drops of Violet Essential Oil

15 Drops of Palmarosa Essential Oil

10 Drops Vetiver Essential Oil

5 Drops Myrrh Essential Oil (refines and smooths skin for older complexions)

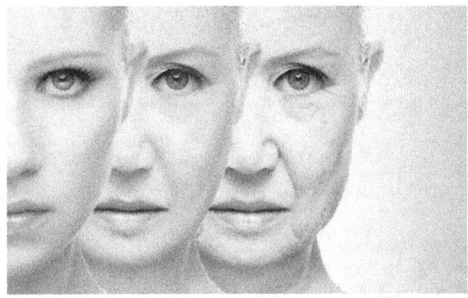

21. Toning for Mature Skin

1/2 Cup Olive Oil

15 Drops Myrtle Essential Oil

15 Drops Naouli Essential Oil

10 Drops Peppermint Essential Oil

10 Drops Grapefruit Essential Oil

22. General Care for Mature Skin

1/2 Cup Coconut Oil

15 Drops Lavender Essential Oil

15 Drops Rosewood Essential Oil

10 Drops Violet Essential Oil

10 Drops Ylang Ylang Essential Oil

23. Oily Mature Skin

1/2 Cup Almond Oil
15 Drops Naouli Essential Oil
10 Drops Bergamot Essential Oil
15 Drops Violet Essential Oil
10 Drops Helichrysum Essential Oil

24. Disinfectant Scrub I

1/2 Cup Coconut Oil
20 Drops Lavender Essential Oil
10 Drops Peppermint Oil
10 Drops Tea Tree Oil
10 Drops Lime Essential Oil

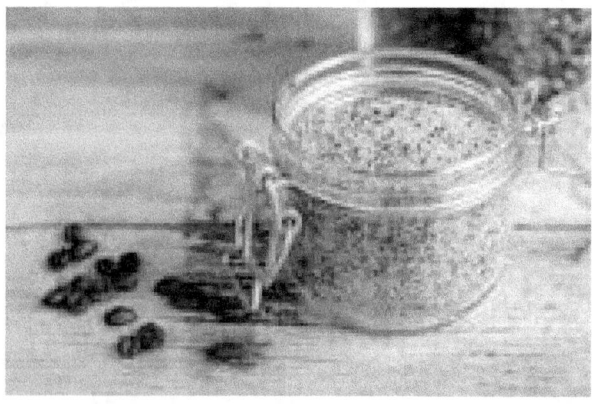

25. Disinfectant and Toning

1/2 Cup Coconut Oil
20 Drops Bergamot Essential Oil
10 Drops Tea Tree Oil
10 Drops Naouli Essential Oil
10 Drops Geranium Essential Oil

26. Disinfectant and Balancing

1/4 Cup Almond Oil
1/4 Cup Coconut Oil
15 Drops Myrtle Essential Oil
15 Drops Patchouli Essential Oil
10 Drops Peppermint Essential Oil
10 Drops Grapefruit Essential Oil

27. Rosacea I

(Don't rub on broken skin or weeping spots)
1/2 Cups Coconut Oil
15 Drops Lavender Essential Oil
15 Drops Rosewood Essential Oil

10 Drops Patchouli Essential Oil
10 Drops Myrtle Essential Oil

28. Rosacea II

1/2 Cup Olive Oil
15 Drops Palmarosa Essential Oil
15 Drops Galbanum Essential Oil
10 Drops Chamomile Essential Oil
10 Drops Tea Tree Essential Oil

29. Exfoliating and Refining I

1/4 Cup roughly ground Coffee grounds
1/4 Cup roughly ground Brown Sugar
1/2 Cup Coconut Oil
15 Drops Grapefruit Essential Oil
15 Drops Peppermint Essential Oil
10 Drops Geranium Essential Oil
10 Drops Helichrysum Essential Oil

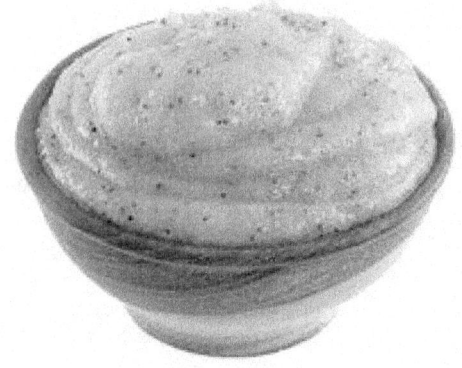

30. Exfoliating and Refining II

1/4 Cup roughly ground Coffee grounds
1/4 Cup roughly ground Brown Sugar
1/2 Cup Coconut Oil
20 Drops Galbanum Essential Oil
10 Drops Pathchouli Essential Oil
10 Drops Grapefruit Essential Oil
10 Drops Lime Essential Oil

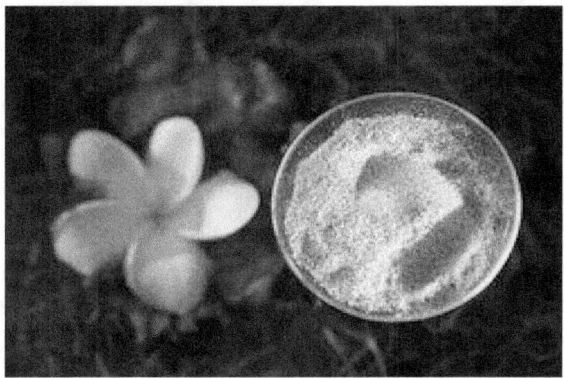

31. Soothing for Mature Skin

1/2 Cup of Coconut Oil

20 Drops of Lavender Essential Oil

15 Drops Palmarosa Essential Oil

15 Drops Rosewood Essential Oil

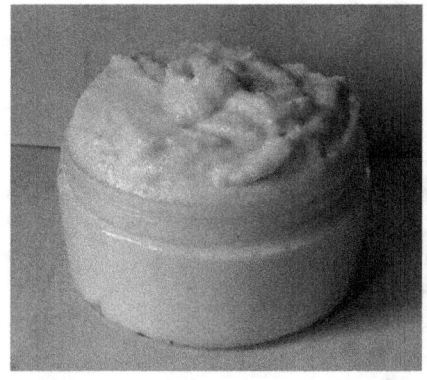

32. Dry Skin for Mature Complexion

1/2 Cup of Olive Oil

15 Drops Chamomile Essential Oil

15 Drops Palmarosa Essential Oil

10 Drops Peppermint Essential Oil

10 Drops Ylang Ylang Essentail Oil

33. Everyday Scrub

1/2 Cup Coconut Oil
10 Drops Chamomile Essential Oil
10 Drops Peppermint Essential Oil
10 Drops Rosewood Essential Oil
10 Drops Grapefruit Essential Oil
10 Drops Palmarosa Essential Oil

34. Mocha Scrub

1/4 Cup Ground Cacao
1/4 Cup Coffee Grinds
1/2 Cup Coconut Oil
15 Drops Rosewood Essential Oil
15 Drops Peppermint Essential Oil
10 Drops Vetiver Essential Oil
10 Drops Bergamot Essential Oil

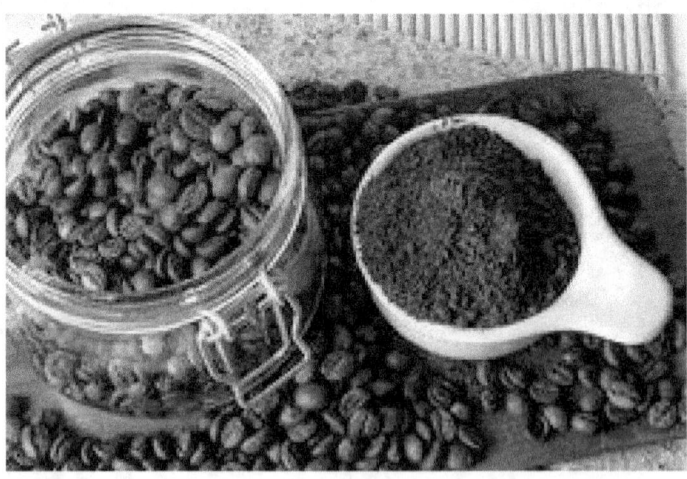

35. Mocha Scrub II

1/4 Cup Ground Cacao
1/4 Cup Coffee Grinds
1/2 Cup Coconut Oil
20 Drops Grapefruit Essential Oil
15 Drops Palmarosa Essential Oil
15 Drops Myrtle Essential Oil

Chapter 3 - Don't stop there...

This is just the start of your hobby. To get a better understanding of essential oils and aromatherapy, join forums where people of like mind share tips, tricks, and knowledge of this most rewarding hobby.

Branch out. Don't just make scrubs. There are so many things you can do with essential oils, and you're ready to look into it. You can make

• Mineral baths
--These can be made of either salts or oatmeal and is good for reducing muscle pains and swelling and softens the skin.

• Facial masks
--Essential oils with their base oils can be mixed with clay powders to tone and cleanse the face.

• Massage oils
--You can combine different essentials with their base oils loosen tight muscles and relax the body.

• Homemade soap
--You can add essential oils to homemade soap to give them an extra kick to cleanse and tone the skin.

• Shampoo Additives
--You can add essential oils to your favorite shampoo to make your hair healthier

• Lotions
--You can either by base lotion or add essential oils to your existing lotion to boost its effectiveness

There are more oils out there

There are over 80 essential oils on the market which can be used for a multitude of purposes and to help treat illnesses.

Resources

There are Ebooks and books you can get at books stores to expand your knowledge on aromatherapy. You can also find forums online with knowledgeable people who can give you advice and recipes. There are websites dedicated to essentials and their uses.

Chapter 4 - Marketing and Selling

When you are comfortable with making your own original recipes and even mixing the ones in the previous chapter, you may wonder if you can break into packaging and selling your own. You can, but there are a few things you will need to get your name out there.

Brand Name

This should be catchy and also tell your potential customers what you are selling. It should be easy to remember and find on the internet.

Labels and Packaging

There are websites out there which can help you design a logo and place the logo on your packaging. You can find the best services when you shop around online.
Look up regulations in your area to see what the requirements are for the ingredients on the label and if you need a disclaimer.

Mixing and Testing

It takes months to formulate, test, and make sure your recipes are safe and effective. You can test the recipes on yourself and your friends and family, if they are willing. Once you have a good base of recipes that work, you are ready to start marketing your products.

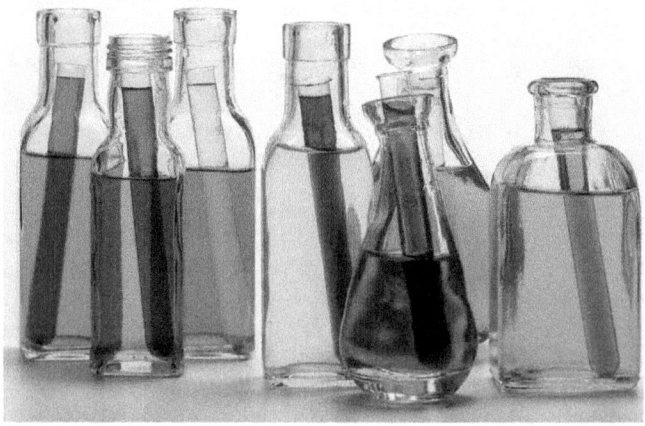

Marketing

No matter what your product is, you have to sell yourself first. You do this by showing the knowledge you have gained through the process. You then build a rapport with your potential customers before you introduce you product line.

Blog

Blogs are a wonderful way to start getting your name out there and showing what you know about essential oils and aromatherapy. Categorized correctly, it makes it easier for you customer base to find in the information. You can also include the process you go through to make your products. As you introduce your products, you can make a blog post with the ingredients and how they work. This will help your customers make a more informed decision.

Social Media

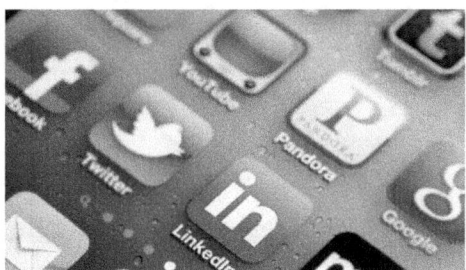

This is a free and effective way to get your name out there. Here are a few things platforms you can use to market your products:

Facebook

Even though they keep changing their algorithm, you can still get your name out there in two ways:

1. Fan Page: With a fan page, you can announce new products, upcoming blog posts and even post info-graphics and small info-memes to keep your customers in the know.

2. Groups: You can start your own group and advertise in it and invite people to join. You can also use this as an online forum to interact further with your customers.

Twitter

You can put small tips and tricks in 140 characters for your customers that like to get quick bursts of information. You can also post info memes and share your blog links here, too.

Instagram

This is where you can really show off your product. You can display product pictures, before and after pictures, and even post informational pictures for your customers to look at and comment on.

Snapchat

You can post short video announcements for new products and answer questions. You can also make sale announcements, too.

YouTube

This may not be an obvious choice for marketing, but making a video on how you make your products will provide a behind-the-scenes way for your customers to find out how products are made. You can also make short informational videos to share on other platforms.

Social Media Marketing Tips

To be effective, there are certain things you need to know about navigating social media:

1. It's social media, not commercial media
--This may sound counter-productive, but sharing little tidbits of your day and what are up to makes you more personable to your customer base. Make about 30% of your media posts about your day.

2. Images attract attention

--Infographics, memes, and collages of your products will draw a customer's eyes to your page and posts. It will increase organic reach and interaction.

3. Interact on other like pages

--Search for other people with interests like yours to engage with and start conversations. Join groups and forums to get your name out there and show your knowledge.

4. Use dashboards

--Use tools like Hootsuite and Buffer to keep all of your social media in one place. These dashboards will let you share your posts over all media without having to go to each one individually. Hootsuite even has tools you can use to receive notifications when someone mentions your name or products without a hashtag.

5. Know your hashtags

--Rite tag is the perfect for making sure your tweets and google+ plus posts will have the best hashtags for the most reach.

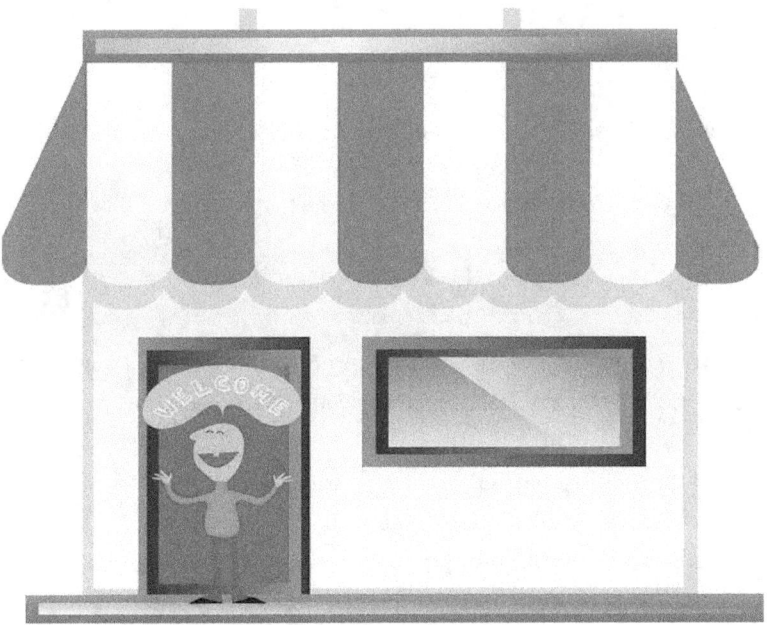

Pricing

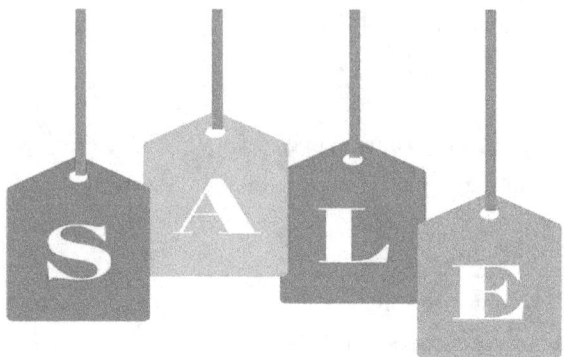

Besides getting the recipes right, the next hardest thing is figuring out how to price your products. Here is what needs to be factored into your final price:

1.   Your labels and packaging,

2.   Shipping,

3.   The individual products you mix in your products,

4.   The time is takes you to formulate and test the product,

5.   Any marketing tools you use to advertise your products,

6.   A portion of your home's mortgage or rent appropriate to the space you use to make your products divided by the number of products you make in a month,

7.   A percentage of the utilities used in the part of your residence,

8.   Finally, the percentage that will constitute your profit.
There are forums online you can go to and ask for more information and formulas to price your products.

Offline Marketing

There are stores out there which are operated by the owners. Before you approach them there are a few things you need to do:

1. Call and introduce yourself and your business. Be professional and polite. Explain the type of products you make and if they would be interested in trying samples. If they say yes, make small samples of the products and have a presentation ready.

2. Your presentation should be quick, concise and informative. It should include how long it would take for you to fill an order for their store and how much stock you have ready to fill that order.

3. Have a cost price for your products. This price should be 10%-20% of the wholesale price (the price of the materials you use).

Open air Markets

You can contact local and out-of-state venues to sell your items.

1. Many cities across the U.S. have monthly markets which will let you set up a booth and sell your products.

2. You can go to Pow-wows to sell your products as well. Native American Pow-wows will also let you set up tents to sell your wares

3. There are also natural health conventions you can register and sell your products.

If you are planning to do any of these, prepare to make more than one trip to these venues. You have to establish a presence and connect with other vendors and venue-goers. Planning on going to several of these each year will expose you to more customers and even customers you've met online will probably be at these events. This will give you a chance to meet them.

Conclusion

I hope this book served you well. I hope the information contained within answered questions and got your creative juices flowing. Never stop making new things. See you next book!